FROM DIAGNOSIS TO CONTROL:

MASTERING DIABETES FOR A BETTER LIFE

DR. MELISSA P. NELSON

TABLE OF CONTENTS

INTRODUCTION

Welcome to "From Diagnosis to Control: Mastering Diabetes for a Better Life." This book is a comprehensive guide that empowers individuals living with diabetes to take charge of their health, embrace a positive mindset, and thrive in their journey towards better diabetes management. Whether you or a loved one has recently been diagnosed with diabetes or have been living with the condition for years, this book is here to offer guidance, support, and valuable insights to help you navigate the challenges and triumphs of diabetes with confidence.

Diabetes is a chronic condition that affects millions of lives worldwide, and its impact reaches far beyond the realm of medicine. We understand that a diabetes diagnosis can be overwhelming, leaving individuals and families with questions, uncertainties, and concerns about the future. However, within every challenge lies an opportunity for growth, learning, and empowerment. This book seeks to provide you with the knowledge, tools, and resources to seize that opportunity and embrace a life of wellness and purpose.

In this journey of understanding and mastering diabetes, we will embark on a transformative exploration of various aspects of diabetes management. We will delve into the different types of diabetes, the underlying causes and risk factors, and the role of insulin and blood sugar regulation. Armed with this knowledge, you will gain a deeper understanding of the condition and lay the foundation for informed decision-making.

As we progress, we will delve into the lifestyle changes that form the pillars of diabetes control. Nutrition plays a pivotal role in managing blood sugar levels, and we will explore how to create balanced meal plans that nourish the body while supporting diabetes management. Physical activity is a powerful tool in diabetes care, and we will discuss how to incorporate regular exercise into daily life to enhance overall well-being.

Embracing a positive mindset is essential in the journey towards better diabetes control. We will address the emotional and psychological aspects of diabetes, providing strategies to cope with stress, manage burnout, and navigate social situations with confidence. By setting realistic goals and celebrating achievements, individuals can foster resilience and build a strong foundation for success.

In this book, we will also delve into the future of diabetes management, exploring the latest advancements in research, technology, and potential cures. Staying informed and engaged in the diabetes community is key to unlocking the full potential of these innovations and accessing valuable support from peers and healthcare professionals.

Ultimately, "From Diagnosis to Control: Mastering Diabetes for a Better Life" seeks to empower you with the knowledge, inspiration, and support needed to navigate the complexities of diabetes with confidence and determination. Together, we will embrace the possibilities that lie ahead, celebrate the triumphs, and find strength in the diabetes community.

Remember, diabetes may be a part of your life, but it does not define you. With the right tools and a positive mindset, you can master diabetes for a better life. Let this book be your companion on this transformative journey, guiding you towards a life of wellness, purpose, and empowerment. Wishing you health, happiness, and success as you embark on this path to better diabetes control and a brighter future.

CHAPTER 1: UNDERSTANDING DIABETES

Diabetes is a chronic medical condition that affects how your body regulates blood sugar levels. There are several types of diabetes, including Type 1, Type 2, and Gestational diabetes.

Types Of Diabetes

Diabetes is a metabolic disorder characterized by elevated blood sugar levels, and there are three main types of diabetes: Type 1, Type 2, and Gestational diabetes. Each type has distinct characteristics, causes, and implications for management.

1. Type 1 Diabetes:

- Type 1 diabetes, also known as insulin-dependent or juvenile diabetes, typically develops during childhood or adolescence.

- It occurs when the immune system mistakenly attacks and destroys the insulin-producing beta cells in the pancreas.

- As a result, the body cannot produce insulin, leading to high blood sugar levels and dependence on external insulin administration.

- The exact cause of Type 1 diabetes is not fully understood, but genetic predisposition and environmental triggers may play a role.

- Individuals with Type 1 diabetes must regularly monitor their blood sugar levels and administer insulin injections or use insulin pumps to manage their condition effectively.

2. Type 2 Diabetes:

- Type 2 diabetes is the most common form of diabetes, accounting for the majority of diabetes cases worldwide.

- It often develops in adulthood, but it is increasingly seen in children and adolescents due to rising obesity rates.

- In Type 2 diabetes, the body's cells become resistant to insulin's effects, and the pancreas may not produce enough insulin to meet the body's needs.

- Lifestyle factors such as sedentary behavior, unhealthy diet, obesity, and genetics play significant roles in its development.

- Initially, Type 2 diabetes can often be managed with lifestyle changes, including weight loss, healthy eating, and regular exercise. However, some people may also require oral medications or insulin therapy over time.

3. Gestational Diabetes:

- Gestational diabetes occurs during pregnancy and affects about 2-10% of pregnant women.

- Hormonal changes during pregnancy can lead to insulin resistance, resulting in elevated blood sugar levels.

- Most women with gestational diabetes can control their blood sugar through dietary changes and physical activity.

- If left unmanaged, gestational diabetes can pose risks to both the mother and the baby, including an increased risk of developing Type 2 diabetes later in life.

- Regular monitoring of blood sugar levels during pregnancy is essential for proper management.

Understanding the different types of diabetes is crucial for early detection, appropriate treatment, and successful management. Proper medical supervision, healthy lifestyle choices, and adherence to treatment plans can help individuals with diabetes lead fulfilling lives while minimizing the risk of complications associated with the condition.

Causes and Risk Factors of Diabetes

Diabetes is a multifactorial condition influenced by a combination of genetic, environmental, and lifestyle factors. Understanding these causes and risk factors is essential for preventing and managing the disease effectively.

Type 1 Diabetes:

Causes: The exact cause of Type 1 diabetes is not fully understood, but it is believed to result from an autoimmune response. The immune system mistakenly attacks and destroys the insulin-producing beta cells in the pancreas, leading to a lack of insulin production.

Risk Factors: Type 1 diabetes is often diagnosed in childhood or adolescence, and family history plays a significant role in its development. Certain genetic markers and exposure to environmental triggers, such as viral infections, may also contribute to the risk.

Type 2 Diabetes:

Causes: Type 2 diabetes develops when the body's cells become resistant to insulin, and the pancreas may not produce enough insulin to compensate for this resistance. Over time, this leads to elevated blood sugar levels.

Risk Factors: Several factors increase the risk of Type 2 diabetes. These include being overweight or obese, leading a sedentary lifestyle, having a family history of diabetes, and belonging to certain ethnic groups (e.g., African American, Hispanic, Asian, or Pacific Islander descent). Age is also a risk factor, with the risk rising after the age of 45.

Gestational Diabetes:

Causes: Gestational diabetes occurs when hormonal changes during pregnancy lead to insulin resistance, similar to Type 2 diabetes. The placenta produces hormones that can interfere with insulin function, resulting in elevated blood sugar levels.

Risk Factors: Women who are overweight, have a family history of diabetes, or have experienced gestational diabetes in previous pregnancies are at higher risk. Advanced maternal age and certain ethnic backgrounds can also increase the likelihood of developing gestational diabetes.

Other Contributing Factors

Prediabetes: Prediabetes is a condition where blood sugar levels are higher than normal but not high enough to be classified as diabetes. People with prediabetes are at an increased risk of developing Type 2 diabetes if lifestyle changes are not made.

Unhealthy Lifestyle: Sedentary behavior, poor dietary habits (high in processed sugars and unhealthy fats), and smoking are associated with an increased risk of diabetes.

Gestational diabetes: Women who have experienced gestational diabetes during pregnancy have a higher risk of developing Type 2 diabetes later in life.

Medical Conditions: Certain medical conditions, such as polycystic ovary syndrome (PCOS) and other hormonal disorders, can increase diabetes risk.

While some risk factors for diabetes, such as age and family history, cannot be changed, adopting a healthy lifestyle can significantly reduce the risk of developing Type 2 diabetes and help manage prediabetes. Regular physical activity, a balanced diet, weight management, and avoiding tobacco use are essential strategies for preventing or delaying the onset of diabetes and its complications.

The Role of Insulin and Blood Sugar Regulation:

Insulin is a hormone produced by the beta cells of the pancreas, and it plays a critical role in regulating blood sugar levels in the body. Blood sugar, also known as blood glucose, is the primary source of energy for the body's cells, and maintaining its levels within a narrow range is essential for overall health.

Insulin's Function:

- After we eat, carbohydrates from the food are broken down into glucose, which enters the bloodstream. The rise in blood sugar levels signals the pancreas to release insulin into the bloodstream.
- Insulin acts as a key that unlocks the body's cells, allowing glucose to enter and be used for energy production or stored as glycogen in the liver and muscles for future use.
- It also facilitates the conversion of excess glucose into fat for long-term energy storage.

Blood Sugar Regulation:

- In a healthy individual, as blood sugar levels rise after a meal, insulin is released to help glucose enter cells and decrease blood sugar levels.
- When blood sugar levels drop, such as between meals or during physical activity, insulin secretion decreases, allowing the body to use stored glucose (glycogen) for energy.

- In cases of low blood sugar, the pancreas releases another hormone called glucagon, which signals the liver to convert stored glycogen back into glucose to raise blood sugar levels.

Diabetes and Blood Sugar Dysregulation:

- In Type 1 diabetes, the immune system mistakenly attacks and destroys the beta cells in the pancreas, resulting in little to no insulin production. Without sufficient insulin, glucose cannot enter cells, leading to high blood sugar levels.

- In Type 2 diabetes, the body's cells become resistant to the effects of insulin, and the pancreas may not produce enough insulin to overcome this resistance. This also results in elevated blood sugar levels.

- Gestational diabetes occurs due to insulin resistance caused by hormonal changes during pregnancy.

Effective blood sugar regulation is essential for overall health, as chronically high blood sugar levels can lead to various complications, such as cardiovascular disease, nerve damage, kidney problems, and eye issues. People with diabetes manage their blood sugar levels through various methods, including insulin therapy (for Type 1 diabetes), oral medications, dietary adjustments, regular physical activity, and monitoring blood sugar levels.

Maintaining blood sugar within the target range is crucial for individuals with diabetes to reduce the risk of complications and achieve better overall well-being. Regular medical check-ups and adherence to prescribed treatment plans are vital for successful diabetes management.

CHAPTER 2: THE DIAGNOSIS JOURNEY

Receiving a diabetes diagnosis is a life-changing moment that can evoke a range of emotions and uncertainties. In this chapter, we explore the emotional impact of a diabetes diagnosis, understanding medical tests and results, and the importance of seeking support and building a healthcare team to navigate the challenges ahead.

The Emotional Impact of a Diabetes Diagnosis

- A diabetes diagnosis can trigger various emotions, including shock, fear, sadness, and even denial. It may require time to come to terms with the condition and its implications on daily life.

- Managing diabetes involves lifestyle changes and constant attention to blood sugar levels, which can be overwhelming and lead to feelings of stress or frustration.

- Addressing emotional well-being is crucial, and seeking support from loved ones, healthcare professionals, or diabetes support groups can help individuals cope with the emotional challenges that come with the diagnosis.

Understanding Medical Tests and Results

- After a diabetes diagnosis, healthcare providers may conduct various medical tests to determine the type of diabetes and its severity.

- Common tests include fasting blood glucose, oral glucose tolerance test (OGTT), hemoglobin A1c (HbA1c), and blood lipid profile. These tests provide valuable information about blood sugar control, overall health, and risk factors for diabetes-related complications.

- Understanding the significance of test results is essential for making informed decisions about treatment and lifestyle adjustments.

Seeking Support and Building a Healthcare Team

- Building a reliable healthcare team is crucial for managing diabetes effectively. This team typically includes primary care physicians, endocrinologists, certified diabetes educators, nutritionists, and other specialists as needed.

- Diabetes self-management requires education and support, and certified diabetes educators can provide valuable guidance on medication, blood sugar monitoring, diet, and exercise.

- Engaging in diabetes support groups or online communities can offer a sense of belonging and valuable insights from others with similar experiences.

- Loved ones' support is vital, as they can play a significant role in providing encouragement and understanding.

Navigating the diagnosis journey requires patience, education, and a positive outlook. By understanding the emotional impact of the diagnosis, learning about medical tests and results, and building a strong healthcare support team, individuals with diabetes can gain confidence in managing their condition and improve their overall well-being. Embracing this journey as an opportunity for growth and empowerment can lead to better long-term health outcomes.

CHAPTER 3: LIFESTYLE CHANGES FOR DIABETES MANAGEMENT

Managing diabetes effectively involves making significant lifestyle changes to achieve optimal blood sugar control and improve overall health. In this chapter, we delve into the importance of diet and nutrition in diabetes control, creating a balanced meal plan, and incorporating regular physical activity into daily life.

Importance of Diet and Nutrition in Diabetes Control

Diet and nutrition play a crucial role in diabetes control, as they directly impact blood sugar levels and overall health. Making informed and healthy food choices can help individuals with diabetes manage their condition effectively and reduce the risk of complications.

Here are some key reasons why diet and nutrition are essential in diabetes control:

1. Blood Sugar Regulation: The primary goal of diabetes management is to keep blood sugar levels within a target range. Foods rich in carbohydrates, such as bread, pasta, rice, and sugary snacks, can cause rapid spikes in blood sugar levels. By monitoring carbohydrate intake and choosing complex carbohydrates with fiber, such as whole grains and vegetables, blood sugar levels can be better regulated.

2. Weight Management: Maintaining a healthy weight is essential for diabetes control, especially for those with Type 2 diabetes. A balanced and nutritious diet can support weight management by providing essential nutrients while controlling calorie intake.

3. Preventing Complications: Uncontrolled diabetes can lead to various complications, including cardiovascular disease, nerve damage, kidney problems, and eye issues. A diet rich in antioxidants, vitamins, and minerals can help protect against oxidative stress and inflammation, reducing the risk of these complications.

4. Improving Insulin Sensitivity: Certain foods, such as those high in unhealthy fats and refined sugars, can increase insulin resistance in the body. On the other hand, a diet rich in healthy fats, lean proteins, and whole foods can improve insulin sensitivity, allowing cells to use glucose more effectively.

5. Supporting Heart Health: People with diabetes are at an increased risk of heart disease. A heart-healthy diet that includes whole grains, fruits, vegetables, and lean proteins can help lower cholesterol levels, reduce blood pressure, and support overall cardiovascular health.

6. Promoting Overall Well-Being: A balanced and nutritious diet can contribute to overall well-being, providing the energy needed for daily activities and promoting a positive outlook on life.

Individuals with diabetes should work with a registered dietitian or healthcare professional to develop a personalized meal plan that suits their specific health needs, lifestyle, and cultural preferences. Consistent monitoring of blood sugar levels and making adjustments to the diet as needed are essential for successful diabetes control.

Remember that diet and nutrition are just one aspect of diabetes management. Regular physical activity, proper medication, and ongoing support from healthcare professionals and loved ones are equally important for achieving optimal blood sugar control and maintaining good health.

Creating a Balanced Meal Plan for Diabetes Control

A balanced meal plan is a key component of diabetes management, helping individuals with diabetes regulate blood sugar levels, maintain a healthy weight, and reduce the risk of complications. A well-designed meal plan focuses on nutrient-rich foods while considering portion sizes and carbohydrate intake.

Here are essential steps to create a balanced meal plan for diabetes:

1. Understanding Carbohydrates:
- Carbohydrates have the most significant impact on blood sugar levels. It is crucial to be mindful of the types and amounts of carbohydrates consumed.

- Focus on complex carbohydrates, such as whole grains, legumes, fruits, and vegetables, which provide fiber and essential nutrients.

- Limit intake of refined carbohydrates, sugary foods, and sweetened beverages, as they can lead to rapid spikes in blood sugar levels.

2. Incorporating Lean Proteins:

- Lean proteins, such as fish, poultry, tofu, and legumes, help stabilize blood sugar levels and provide essential amino acids for tissue repair and maintenance.

- Including proteins in meals can also help increase satiety and reduce the overall glycemic impact of the meal.

3. Emphasizing Healthy Fats:

- Healthy fats, such as those found in avocados, nuts, seeds, and olive oil, play a role in heart health and can help slow the absorption of carbohydrates, stabilizing blood sugar levels.

- Moderation is key since fats are calorie-dense.

4. Portion Control:

- Monitoring portion sizes is crucial for diabetes management and weight control.

- Using smaller plates and measuring portion sizes can help avoid overeating.

5. Spreading Meals Throughout the Day:

- Distributing meals evenly throughout the day can help regulate blood sugar levels and prevent large fluctuations.

- Including healthy snacks between meals can help maintain energy levels and prevent overeating during main meals.

6. Monitoring Glycemic Index (GI):

- The glycemic index measures how quickly foods raise blood sugar levels. Foods with a low GI have a slower impact on blood sugar, providing more stable energy levels.

- Combining low GI foods with higher GI foods can help moderate the overall glycemic impact of a meal.

7. Personalization and Flexibility:

- Everyone's dietary needs and preferences are unique. A balanced meal plan should be personalized to suit individual health goals and cultural preferences.

- Flexibility allows for occasional indulgences without compromising overall diabetes control.

It is crucial for individuals with diabetes to work with a registered dietitian or healthcare professional to develop a personalized meal plan. Regular monitoring of blood sugar levels and adjustments to the meal plan based on individual responses are essential for successful diabetes management.

Creating a balanced meal plan empowers individuals with diabetes to make healthy food choices, manage their condition effectively, and achieve overall well-being. By combining nutritious foods, portion control, and consistent monitoring, individuals can take charge of their health and enjoy a fulfilling and balanced lifestyle.

Incorporating Regular Physical Activity into Daily Life for Diabetes Management

Regular physical activity is a vital aspect of diabetes management, offering numerous health benefits and helping individuals with diabetes improve blood sugar control and overall well-being. Engaging in regular exercise can enhance insulin sensitivity, reduce insulin resistance, and support weight management.

Here are key strategies for incorporating physical activity into daily life:

1. Choose Activities You Enjoy:

- Find physical activities that you enjoy, whether it's walking, dancing, swimming, cycling, yoga, or playing a sport.

- When you enjoy an activity, it becomes easier to stay motivated and make it a regular part of your daily routine.

2. Start Slowly and Gradually Increase:

- If you're new to exercise or have been inactive for a while, start slowly and gradually increase the intensity and duration of your activities.

- Aim for at least 150 minutes of moderate-intensity aerobic activity or 75 minutes of vigorous-intensity aerobic activity per week, spread throughout the week.

3. Incorporate Strength Training:

- Strength training, such as weightlifting or resistance exercises, helps build muscle mass, which can improve insulin sensitivity and enhance overall metabolism.

- Include strength training exercises at least two days a week, targeting major muscle groups.

4. Be Active Throughout the Day:

- Look for opportunities to be active throughout the day, such as taking short walks during breaks, using stairs instead of elevators, or doing houschold chores that require physical effort.

- Even brief bursts of activity can add up and contribute to improved health.

5. Stay Safe and Monitor Blood Sugar Levels:

- Consult your healthcare provider before starting a new exercise regimen, especially if you have any underlying health conditions.

- Monitor your blood sugar levels before, during, and after exercise to understand how physical activity affects your body.

6. Buddy Up for Motivation:

- Exercising with a friend or family member can be fun and motivating. Having a workout buddy can help you stay accountable and committed to your fitness goals.

7. Set Realistic Goals:

- Set achievable and realistic goals for your physical activity. Gradual progress is better than pushing yourself too hard and risking injury.

- Celebrate your achievements, no matter how small, to stay motivated and positive.

Regular physical activity not only helps manage blood sugar levels but also improves cardiovascular health, reduces stress, and boosts overall energy and well-being. Remember that any amount of activity is better than none, so find ways to incorporate movement into your daily life and make exercise a rewarding and enjoyable part of your diabetes management plan.

CHAPTER 4: MONITORING BLOOD SUGAR LEVELS

Monitoring blood sugar levels is a critical aspect of diabetes management, providing valuable insights into how various factors affect blood glucose levels. In this chapter, we explore different methods of blood sugar monitoring, interpreting blood sugar readings, and effective ways to track and manage blood sugar fluctuations.

Different Methods of Blood Sugar Monitoring

Blood sugar monitoring is a critical aspect of diabetes management, allowing individuals to track their blood glucose levels and make informed decisions about their treatment and lifestyle choices. Several methods are available for monitoring blood sugar, each with its benefits and considerations. Here are the different methods of blood sugar monitoring:

Self-Monitoring Blood Glucose (SMBG):
 - SMBG is the most common method of blood sugar monitoring and involves using a blood glucose meter at home.

- To perform SMBG, a small drop of blood is obtained by pricking the fingertip with a lancet. The blood is then applied to a test strip inserted into the meter.

- The meter quickly measures the blood glucose level, which is displayed on the screen.

- SMBG allows individuals to check their blood sugar at various times throughout the day, such as before and after meals or exercise, and to make real-time adjustments to their diabetes management plan.

Continuous Glucose Monitoring (CGM):

- CGM is a more advanced method of blood sugar monitoring that provides continuous data throughout the day and night.

- A CGM device is usually worn on the skin and contains a small sensor inserted under the skin to measure interstitial fluid glucose levels.

- The device transmits blood glucose readings to a receiver or smartphone, allowing users to see real-time trends, glucose patterns, and alarms for high or low blood sugar levels.

- CGM provides valuable insights into blood sugar fluctuations and helps individuals identify trends and patterns, leading to better diabetes management.

Flash Glucose Monitoring:

- Flash glucose monitoring is similar to CGM but does not provide continuous real-time data. Instead, users scan the sensor with a reader or smartphone to obtain a glucose reading.

- This method is less intrusive than SMBG as it does not require finger pricks, but it offers data in the form of a "snapshot" rather than continuous monitoring.

Continuous Interstitial Glucose Monitoring (CIGM):

- CIGM is an emerging method that combines features of both CGM and flash glucose monitoring.

- It provides continuous data like CGM but does not require regular scanning. Instead, users wear a device that automatically logs the glucose data and allows for retrospective analysis.

Each method of blood sugar monitoring has its advantages and limitations. SMBG provides immediate feedback and is suitable for most individuals with diabetes. CGM offers continuous data and real-time insights, making it beneficial for those requiring intensive glucose management or at risk of severe blood sugar fluctuations.

Choosing the most appropriate method depends on individual preferences, lifestyle, and healthcare provider recommendations. Consistent and accurate blood sugar monitoring is essential for effective diabetes management, enabling individuals to make timely adjustments to their treatment plan and maintain stable blood glucose levels for improved overall health.

Interpreting Blood Sugar Readings

Interpreting blood sugar readings is a critical skill for individuals with diabetes as it provides valuable insights into their blood glucose levels and overall diabetes management. Understanding blood sugar readings helps individuals make informed decisions about medication, diet, physical activity, and lifestyle adjustments.

Here's a guide to interpreting blood sugar readings:

Fasting Blood Sugar:

- Fasting blood sugar is measured after an overnight fast, typically eight hours without eating.

- A normal fasting blood sugar level is usually between 70-100 mg/dL (3.9-5.6 mmol/L).

- Higher readings may indicate poor overnight blood sugar control and could be a sign of uncontrolled diabetes or prediabetes.

Postprandial Blood Sugar:
- Postprandial blood sugar is measured one to two hours after a meal.

- A healthy postprandial reading is generally below 140 mg/dL (7.8 mmol/L) for most individuals with diabetes.

- Keeping postprandial blood sugar levels in the target range helps prevent spikes and reduce the risk of complications.

Hemoglobin A1c (HbA1c):
- HbA1c provides an average blood sugar level over the past two to three months, indicating long-term glucose control.

- A target HbA1c level for most individuals with diabetes is below 7% (53 mmol/mol).

- Higher HbA1c levels suggest poorer overall diabetes management and may require adjustments to the treatment plan.

Patterns and Trends:
- Monitoring blood sugar readings over time helps identify patterns and trends.
- Tracking blood sugar levels before and after meals, before bedtime, and during specific activities can reveal how certain factors affect blood glucose levels.
- Consistent patterns of high or low readings may indicate the need for adjustments in medication, meal planning, or physical activity routines.

Hypoglycemia:
- Hypoglycemia, or low blood sugar, is when blood sugar levels drop below 70 mg/dL (3.9 mmol/L).

- Symptoms of hypoglycemia include shakiness, dizziness, sweating, confusion, and rapid heartbeat.

- Promptly treating hypoglycemia with fast-acting carbohydrates is essential to raise blood sugar levels to a safe range.

Hyperglycemia:

- Hyperglycemia, or high blood sugar, is when blood sugar levels exceed the target range.

- Symptoms of hyperglycemia include frequent urination, excessive thirst, fatigue, and blurred vision.

- Addressing hyperglycemia may involve adjusting medication, increasing physical activity, or reevaluating dietary choices.

Interpreting blood sugar readings requires continuous monitoring, record-keeping, and collaboration with healthcare professionals. Regular communication with a healthcare team can help individuals understand their blood sugar trends, make necessary adjustments, and develop a personalized diabetes management plan to achieve optimal blood sugar control and improve overall health.

Tracking and Managing Blood Sugar Fluctuations

Tracking and managing blood sugar fluctuations is essential for individuals with diabetes to maintain optimal blood glucose control and prevent complications. Consistent monitoring and analysis of blood sugar readings help identify patterns, triggers, and trends, enabling individuals to make informed decisions and adjustments to their diabetes management plan.

Here are key strategies for tracking and managing blood sugar fluctuations:

Keep a Blood Sugar Log:
  - Maintain a blood sugar logbook to record daily glucose readings, insulin doses, medication, meals, physical activity, and any significant events affecting blood sugar levels.

  - A logbook helps identify patterns, such as high or low blood sugar levels at specific times of the day or after certain meals, and supports better diabetes management.

Use Blood Glucose Meters or Continuous Glucose Monitoring (CGM) Systems:
  - Regular self-monitoring of blood glucose (SMBG) using a blood glucose meter or continuous glucose monitoring (CGM) provides real-time data on blood sugar fluctuations.

- CGM offers continuous monitoring, helping individuals identify trends and patterns, and provides alerts for high or low blood sugar levels.

Identify Triggers and Patterns:
  - Analyze blood sugar data over time to identify patterns and factors that contribute to blood sugar fluctuations.

  - Common triggers may include specific foods, physical activity, stress, illness, or changes in medication.

Adjust Meal Plans and Carbohydrate Intake:
  - Based on blood sugar trends, work with a registered dietitian to adjust meal plans and manage carbohydrate intake.

  - Consistent carbohydrate counting can help individuals match insulin doses to food intake, promoting better blood sugar control.

Monitor Medication and Insulin Regimen:
  - Regularly review and adjust medication and insulin regimens as needed, based on blood sugar trends and in consultation with healthcare professionals.

- Individualized insulin therapy can help manage blood sugar fluctuations and achieve target levels.

Address Hypoglycemia and Hyperglycemia:

- Promptly treat hypoglycemia (low blood sugar) with fast-acting carbohydrates to raise blood sugar levels to a safe range.

- Address hyperglycemia (high blood sugar) by adjusting insulin doses, increasing physical activity, or reevaluating dietary choices.

Regular Follow-Ups with Healthcare Professionals:

- Schedule regular check-ups and follow-ups with healthcare professionals to review blood sugar trends and make necessary adjustments to the diabetes management plan.

Lifestyle Modifications:

- Incorporate regular physical activity into daily routines to improve insulin sensitivity and support blood sugar control.

- Manage stress through relaxation techniques, such as meditation or yoga, as stress can impact blood sugar levels.

Consistent tracking and management of blood sugar fluctuations empower individuals with diabetes to take charge of their health and make proactive decisions to achieve optimal diabetes control. Effective blood sugar management, in combination with a balanced diet, regular exercise, and adherence to the prescribed treatment plan, can help individuals with diabetes lead fulfilling lives while reducing the risk of complications associated with the condition.

CHAPTER 5: MEDICATIONS AND INSULIN MANAGEMENT

Effective management of diabetes often involves the use of medications and insulin therapy to achieve optimal blood sugar control. In this chapter, we explore common diabetes medications and their functions, insulin therapy including types, delivery methods, and dosage, as well as the importance of adhering to medication schedules and making necessary adjustments.

Common Diabetes Medications and Their Functions

Diabetes medications are essential tools for managing blood sugar levels and preventing complications associated with the condition. Each type of medication works in different ways to help control glucose levels and improve insulin sensitivity. Here are some common diabetes medications and their functions:

Metformin:

Function: Metformin is a widely prescribed oral medication for Type 2 diabetes.

Mechanism: It works by reducing the liver's production of glucose and enhancing insulin sensitivity in the body's cells, allowing them to use glucose more effectively.

Benefits: Metformin is often the first-line treatment for Type 2 diabetes and helps improve blood sugar control and lower HbA1c levels.

Sulfonylureas:

Function: Sulfonylureas are oral medications used to treat Type 2 diabetes.

Mechanism: They stimulate the pancreas to produce more insulin, increasing insulin levels in the bloodstream.

Benefits: Sulfonylureas can quickly lower blood sugar levels and are effective when lifestyle changes and metformin alone are insufficient for diabetes control.

DPP-4 Inhibitors (Gliptins):

Function: DPP-4 inhibitors are oral medications used in Type 2 diabetes.

Mechanism: They work by blocking the enzyme DPP-4, which breaks down certain gut hormones involved in glucose regulation (GLP-1 and GIP). This leads to increased insulin secretion and reduced glucagon production, ultimately lowering blood sugar levels.

Benefits: DPP-4 inhibitors are well-tolerated and can be used as monotherapy or in combination with other diabetes medications.

GLP-1 Receptor Agonists (Incretin Mimetics):

Function: GLP-1 receptor agonists are injectable medications for Type 2 diabetes.

Mechanism: They mimic the action of the hormone GLP-1, which stimulates insulin secretion, slows gastric emptying, and reduces appetite.

Benefits: GLP-1 receptor agonists can improve blood sugar control, promote weight loss, and have a low risk of hypoglycemia.

SGLT2 Inhibitors:

Function: SGLT2 inhibitors are oral medications used in Type 2 diabetes.

Mechanism: They work by blocking the SGLT2 protein in the kidneys, which reduces the reabsorption of glucose and increases glucose excretion in the urine.

Benefits: SGLT2 inhibitors lower blood sugar levels independently of insulin, promote weight loss, and can have cardiovascular benefits.

It is essential to note that each person's response to diabetes medications may vary. Healthcare providers consider individual health status, diabetes type, and other factors to determine the most appropriate medication regimen. Combining medication with a healthy diet, regular physical activity, and blood sugar monitoring helps individuals achieve better blood sugar control and improve their overall health and quality of life.

Insulin Therapy: Types, Delivery Methods, and Dosage

Insulin therapy plays a crucial role in managing diabetes, particularly for individuals with Type 1 diabetes and some with Type 2 diabetes. Insulin is a hormone that helps regulate blood sugar levels by facilitating the uptake of glucose by cells. Here's an overview of insulin therapy, including the different types of insulin, delivery methods, and dosage considerations:

Types of Insulin:

- Rapid-Acting Insulin: Rapid-acting insulin, such as insulin lispro, aspart, or glulisine, starts working within 15 minutes of injection and peaks around 1 to 2 hours after injection. It is typically taken before meals to cover the rise in blood sugar after eating.

- Short-Acting (Regular) Insulin: Regular insulin begins working within 30 minutes and peaks between 2 to 3 hours after injection. It is usually taken 30 minutes before meals to manage post-meal blood sugar levels.

- Intermediate-Acting Insulin: Intermediate-acting insulin, like NPH insulin, starts working within 1 to 2 hours after injection and peaks around 4 to 12 hours. It is often taken twice daily to cover blood sugar levels between meals and during the night.

- Long-Acting Insulin: Long-acting insulin, such as insulin glargine or insulin detemir, has a slow and steady release over an extended period, usually lasting up to 24 hours. It is taken once or twice daily to provide basal insulin coverage, maintaining blood sugar levels between meals and overnight.

Delivery Methods:

 - Insulin Pens: Insulin pens are a popular and convenient way to administer insulin. They come prefilled with insulin cartridges or as disposable pens with replaceable insulin cartridges. Insulin pens allow for easy dose adjustment and discreet use.

 - Insulin Syringes: Insulin can also be administered using traditional insulin syringes, which require drawing the desired dose from a vial of insulin. Although syringes require more manual handling, they offer flexibility in dosing.

 - Insulin Pumps: Insulin pumps are small devices that deliver a continuous supply of rapid-acting insulin throughout the day through a small catheter placed under the skin. Users can also give additional insulin doses before meals, replicating the function of a healthy pancreas more closely.

Dosage Considerations:

- Individualized Dosing: Insulin dosages are tailored to each person's specific needs, considering factors such as age, weight, activity level, blood sugar targets, and response to insulin.

- Basal and Bolus Insulin: Insulin therapy often involves a combination of basal insulin (long-acting) to provide a steady background insulin level and bolus insulin (rapid-acting) to cover blood sugar spikes after meals.

- Adjusting Insulin Doses: Insulin dosages may need to be adjusted based on blood sugar monitoring, carbohydrate intake, physical activity, illness, and other factors that can affect blood sugar levels.

Individuals with diabetes work closely with their healthcare team to determine the most suitable insulin regimen, delivery method, and dosages for effective blood sugar management. Adherence to prescribed insulin therapy and regular blood sugar monitoring are essential components of successful diabetes management, helping individuals achieve optimal blood sugar control and improve their overall health and well-being.

Adhering to Medication Schedules and Adjustments

Adherence to medication schedules is crucial for individuals with diabetes to effectively manage their condition and achieve optimal blood sugar control. It involves taking medications as prescribed by healthcare professionals, following the recommended dosage and timing, and making necessary adjustments when needed.

Here's why adhering to medication schedules and making adjustments is vital for diabetes management:

Blood Sugar Control:

 - Consistent adherence to medication schedules helps maintain stable blood sugar levels, preventing dangerous fluctuations and reducing the risk of hyperglycemia (high blood sugar) and hypoglycemia (low blood sugar).
 - Properly managed blood sugar levels lower the risk of long-term complications associated with diabetes, such as cardiovascular disease, nerve damage, kidney problems, and vision issues.

Treatment Effectiveness:

- Following prescribed medication schedules ensures that the medications can work as intended, delivering the expected benefits for blood sugar control and overall health.

- Skipping doses or not taking medications as directed may result in suboptimal blood sugar management, leading to potential health complications.

Medication Dosage and Timing Adjustments:

- Adherence to medication schedules enables healthcare providers to assess the effectiveness of the current treatment plan and make necessary adjustments.

- Regular monitoring of blood sugar levels helps healthcare professionals determine whether medication dosages need to be modified to achieve target blood sugar levels.

Lifestyle Changes:

- Medication schedules may need to be adjusted when individuals make significant lifestyle changes, such as changes in diet, physical activity, or work routine.

- Open communication with healthcare providers about lifestyle changes can ensure appropriate adjustments are made to the medication regimen.

Avoiding Medication Errors:

- Adhering to medication schedules reduces the risk of medication errors, such as double dosing or missing doses, which can lead to adverse effects on blood sugar levels and health.

Individualized Diabetes Management:

- Adherence to medication schedules allows healthcare providers to tailor diabetes management plans to each individual's specific needs and goals.
- Adjustments to medication schedules can be personalized based on lifestyle, health status, and individual responses to medications.

To improve adherence to medication schedules and adjustments:

- Establish a daily routine for taking medications, making it easier to remember and incorporate into daily life.
- Use medication organizers or reminders on smartphones to prompt timely dosing.
- Communicate openly with healthcare providers about any challenges faced with adherence, potential side effects, or difficulties with medication administration.

Ultimately, adhering to medication schedules and making necessary adjustments empowers individuals with diabetes to take control of their health and successfully manage their condition. By working closely with healthcare professionals and committing to their prescribed treatment plans, individuals can achieve better blood sugar control, reduce the risk of complications, and enjoy a higher quality of life.

CHAPTER 6: COPING WITH DIABETES-RELATED CHALLENGES

Living with diabetes can present various challenges that extend beyond the physical aspects of managing the condition. In this chapter, we explore coping strategies to address the psychological and emotional aspects of diabetes, dealing with diabetes-related stress and burnout, and handling social situations while managing peer pressure.

Addressing Psychological and Emotional Aspects of Diabetes

Living with diabetes involves not only managing the physical aspects of the condition but also addressing the psychological and emotional impact it can have on individuals. Diabetes can lead to a range of emotions, from frustration and anxiety to guilt and fear, due to the daily challenges of blood sugar control, lifestyle changes, and the potential long-term complications.

Here are some strategies to address the psychological and emotional aspects of diabetes:

Education and Understanding:

- Learning about diabetes, its management, and potential complications can help individuals gain a better understanding of the condition, which can reduce anxiety and fear.

- Staying informed empowers individuals to take an active role in their diabetes management, leading to a sense of control over the condition.

Seeking Support:

- Connecting with others who have diabetes through support groups or online forums can provide a sense of camaraderie and empathy.

- Sharing experiences and feelings with others who understand the challenges of diabetes can help individuals feel less alone in their journey.

Professional Counseling or Therapy:

- Diabetes-related stress and emotional challenges may benefit from professional counseling or therapy.

- Talking to a mental health professional can provide a safe space to explore emotions, develop coping strategies, and manage diabetes-related concerns effectively.

Setting Realistic Goals:

- Setting achievable and realistic goals for blood sugar control and diabetes management can reduce feelings of frustration and failure.

- Celebrating small victories and progress can boost motivation and overall emotional well-being.

Mindfulness and Stress Management:

- Practicing mindfulness and stress-reducing techniques, such as meditation, deep breathing exercises, or yoga, can help manage anxiety and emotional stress.

- Engaging in hobbies or activities that bring joy and relaxation can also contribute to emotional well-being.

Open Communication:

- Talking openly about diabetes with family, friends, and coworkers can foster understanding and support.

- Communicating needs and concerns can help others provide the necessary support and reduce any unnecessary pressure or misunderstandings.

Recognizing and Managing Burnout:

- Diabetes management can be challenging, and individuals may experience burnout at times.

- Recognizing signs of burnout, such as exhaustion or lack of motivation, and taking time for self-care can prevent emotional exhaustion.

Addressing the psychological and emotional aspects of diabetes is an essential part of overall diabetes management. It involves acknowledging and accepting one's emotions while actively seeking support, information, and coping mechanisms. Embracing a positive mindset and being proactive in emotional well-being can enhance resilience and lead to a better quality of life for individuals living with diabetes. Remember that it is okay to seek help when needed and that emotional well-being is an essential component of living well with diabetes.

Dealing with Diabetes-Related Stress and Burnout

Living with diabetes can sometimes lead to stress and burnout due to the ongoing demands of managing the condition. Diabetes-related stress may arise from the constant need to monitor blood sugar levels, adhere to medication regimens, make dietary adjustments, and cope with potential complications. Burnout can result from feeling overwhelmed, exhausted, and emotionally drained by the daily responsibilities of diabetes management.

Here are some strategies to cope with diabetes-related stress and prevent burnout:

Seek Support:

- Reach out to family, friends, or support groups to share your feelings and experiences related to diabetes.

- Connecting with others who understand the challenges of diabetes can provide empathy, encouragement, and practical advice.

Set Realistic Goals:

- Break down diabetes management tasks into manageable steps and set realistic goals.

- Celebrate small achievements and progress, as it can boost motivation and reduce feelings of overwhelm.

Practice Stress-Reduction Techniques:

- Engage in stress-reduction activities such as meditation, deep breathing exercises, yoga, or spending time in nature.

- Regularly incorporating these practices into daily life can help manage stress and improve emotional well-being.

Take Breaks and Rest:

- Allow yourself to take breaks and rest when needed. Diabetes management can be demanding, and self-care is essential for preventing burnout.

- Prioritize sleep and ensure you are getting enough rest to recharge both physically and emotionally.

Seek Professional Help:

- If diabetes-related stress becomes overwhelming, consider seeking support from a mental health professional.

- Professional counseling or therapy can provide a safe space to explore emotions, develop coping strategies, and manage stress more effectively.

Engage in Hobbies and Relaxation:

- Engaging in hobbies or activities that bring joy and relaxation can provide a welcome distraction from diabetes-related stress.

- Finding time for enjoyable activities helps create a balanced and fulfilling life.

Adjust Diabetes Management Plan:

- Work with your healthcare team to review your diabetes management plan and explore potential adjustments.

- Discuss concerns or challenges you face in managing diabetes, as they may lead to changes in medication, meal planning, or other aspects of your care.

Practice Mindfulness:
- Mindfulness involves staying present in the moment and acknowledging your feelings without judgment.
- Practicing mindfulness can help you manage stress and prevent negative emotions from becoming overwhelming.

Remember that experiencing stress and occasional burnout is normal, but it is essential to address these feelings and take proactive steps to manage them. Seeking support, practicing self-care, and making lifestyle adjustments can enhance resilience and help individuals better cope with diabetes-related stress, leading to improved overall well-being and a more positive approach to diabetes management.

Handling Social Situations and Managing Peer Pressure with Diabetes

Social situations can present unique challenges for individuals with diabetes, particularly when it comes to managing food choices, insulin dosing, and handling peer pressure related to diabetes management.

Here are some strategies to navigate social settings confidently while effectively managing diabetes:

Educate and Advocate:
- Educate friends, family, and peers about diabetes, its management, and the importance of adhering to a diabetes-friendly lifestyle.
- Be open about your diabetes needs and advocate for your health, helping others understand your dietary and medication requirements.

Plan Ahead:
- Before attending social events, plan your meals and insulin dosing accordingly.
- Bring diabetes-friendly snacks or dishes to gatherings, ensuring you have suitable options available.

Communicate with Hosts:
- If attending an event where food will be served, communicate with the hosts about your dietary needs.
- Sharing your preferences or restrictions can help hosts accommodate your needs.

Be Confident:

- Stay confident in managing your diabetes and make decisions based on your health needs.

- Don't be afraid to decline food or beverages that don't align with your diabetes management plan.

Set Boundaries:

- Establish personal boundaries regarding your diabetes management and communicate them assertively.

- Let others know what you are comfortable discussing or sharing regarding your condition.

Engage Supportive Friends:

- Surround yourself with friends who are supportive and understanding of your diabetes management.

- Trusted friends can help advocate for your needs in social settings.

Be Prepared for Peer Pressure:

- Be prepared to handle peer pressure related to food choices, alcohol consumption, or skipping medication.

- Practice assertive responses to decline offers that do not align with your diabetes management goals.

Focus on the Experience:

- Instead of solely focusing on food, engage in the social experience, conversations, and activities.

- Shifting the focus can help minimize feelings of exclusion or pressure related to food choices.

Seek Online Support:

- Join online diabetes support groups or communities where individuals share their experiences and strategies for managing diabetes in social settings.

- Learning from others' experiences can be empowering and provide practical tips for handling social situations.

Remember that diabetes management is a priority for your health and well-being. Managing diabetes effectively requires balance, confidence, and the ability to advocate for yourself in social settings. Embrace open communication and planning to ensure that social events remain enjoyable and supportive of your diabetes management goals. With practice and support, handling social situations with diabetes becomes more manageable, empowering you to live a fulfilling life while managing your health effectively.

CHAPTER 7: PREVENTING DIABETES COMPLICATIONS

Preventing diabetes complications is essential for maintaining overall health and well-being. In this chapter, we explore the potential complications of uncontrolled diabetes, provide tips for managing and reducing the risk of complications, and emphasize the importance of regular health screenings and check-ups.

Understanding Potential Complications of Uncontrolled Diabetes

Uncontrolled diabetes can lead to a range of serious complications that affect various parts of the body. These complications arise when consistently high blood sugar levels, or hyperglycemia, cause damage to blood vessels and nerves over time.

Here are some of the potential complications of uncontrolled diabetes:

Cardiovascular Complications:

- Heart Disease: Uncontrolled diabetes increases the risk of heart disease and coronary artery disease. High blood sugar levels can damage blood vessels, leading to atherosclerosis (narrowing and hardening of arteries) and an increased risk of heart attacks and chest pain (angina).

- Stroke: Diabetes raises the risk of stroke by damaging blood vessels and increasing the likelihood of blood clots in the brain.

Neuropathy:

- Peripheral Neuropathy: Elevated blood sugar levels can damage nerves in the extremities, leading to peripheral neuropathy. Symptoms may include pain, tingling, numbness, and weakness in the hands and feet.

- Autonomic Neuropathy: Diabetes can affect the autonomic nerves, which control vital functions such as heart rate, blood pressure, digestion, and bladder function. Autonomic neuropathy can lead to various symptoms, including dizziness, fainting, digestive issues, and problems with bladder control.

Nephropathy:

- Diabetic Nephropathy: Uncontrolled diabetes can damage the small blood vessels in the kidneys, leading to diabetic nephropathy. This condition can progress to chronic kidney disease (CKD) and, in severe cases, kidney failure, necessitating dialysis or a kidney transplant.

Retinopathy:

- Diabetic Retinopathy: Prolonged high blood sugar levels can damage the blood vessels in the retina, the light-sensitive tissue at the back of the eye. Diabetic retinopathy can cause vision problems, including blurred vision, floaters, and, in severe cases, vision loss.

Foot Complications:

- Peripheral Arterial Disease: Diabetes can lead to poor circulation in the legs and feet, increasing the risk of peripheral arterial disease (PAD). PAD may result in pain, infections, and slow-healing foot ulcers.

- Diabetic Foot Ulcers: Nerve damage and reduced blood flow can lead to foot ulcers, which, if left untreated, may become infected and potentially lead to gangrene, requiring amputation.

Infections:

- Uncontrolled diabetes weakens the immune system, making individuals more susceptible to infections, particularly skin infections, urinary tract infections (UTIs), and yeast infections.

It is essential for individuals with diabetes to prioritize blood sugar control through medication adherence, a balanced diet, regular exercise, and regular medical check-ups. By effectively managing diabetes, individuals can significantly reduce the risk of complications and maintain better overall health and well-being. Early detection and appropriate management of complications are critical for preventing further progression and preserving quality of life for individuals living with diabetes.

Tips for Managing and Reducing the Risk of Complications

Effectively managing diabetes is essential for reducing the risk of complications and maintaining overall health. By adopting a proactive approach to diabetes management, individuals can significantly lower the likelihood of diabetes-related complications. Here are some essential tips for managing and reducing the risk of complications:

Blood Sugar Control:

- Monitor Blood Sugar: Regularly check blood sugar levels as directed by healthcare professionals. Monitoring helps identify trends and make necessary adjustments to medication, diet, and lifestyle.

- Adhere to Medication Regimen: Take prescribed medications, including insulin and oral medications, as directed by healthcare providers. Follow the recommended dosages and timing.

- Monitor Carbohydrate Intake: Be mindful of carbohydrate consumption, as it directly impacts blood sugar levels. Plan meals to include a balanced combination of carbohydrates, proteins, and healthy fats.

Healthy Diet:

- Choose Nutrient-Rich Foods: Opt for whole grains, lean proteins, fruits, vegetables, and healthy fats in your diet.

- Limit Sugary and Processed Foods: Minimize intake of sugary beverages, sweets, and processed foods high in unhealthy fats and added sugars.

Regular Physical Activity:

- Engage in Regular Exercise: Incorporate physical activity into your daily routine. Aim for at least 150 minutes of moderate-intensity aerobic activity per week, such as brisk walking, swimming, or cycling.

- Include Strength Training: Add strength training exercises at least twice a week to build muscle and improve overall fitness.

Blood Pressure and Cholesterol Management:

- Monitor Blood Pressure: Regularly check blood pressure and follow your healthcare provider's recommendations for maintaining healthy levels.

- Manage Cholesterol: Monitor cholesterol levels and work with healthcare professionals to manage them through lifestyle changes and, if necessary, medication.

Avoid Smoking:

- Quit Smoking: If you smoke, quit as soon as possible. Smoking exacerbates the complications associated with diabetes and increases the risk of cardiovascular diseases.

Regular Health Check-Ups:

- Schedule Regular Check-Ups: Visit your healthcare provider regularly for comprehensive diabetes care and overall health assessments.

- Screenings and Tests: Undergo recommended screenings for complications such as retinopathy, nephropathy, neuropathy, and cardiovascular disease.

Stress Management:

- Practice Stress-Reduction Techniques: Engage in activities that reduce stress, such as meditation, deep breathing exercises, yoga, or spending time in nature.

- Find Stress-Relieving Hobbies: Engage in hobbies or activities that bring joy and relaxation.

Diabetes Education and Support:

- Stay Informed: Continuously educate yourself about diabetes management, new treatment options, and potential complications.

- Join Support Groups: Participate in diabetes support groups or online communities to connect with others who share similar experiences and challenges.

By incorporating these tips into your daily life, you can actively manage diabetes and reduce the risk of complications. Remember that diabetes management is a journey that requires commitment, support, and ongoing communication with healthcare professionals. Prioritizing your health through effective diabetes management contributes to a better quality of life and reduces the impact of diabetes-related complications on your overall well-being.

Regular Health Screenings and Check-ups

Regular health screenings and check-ups are essential components of diabetes management and overall health maintenance. These routine examinations allow healthcare professionals to monitor your diabetes, detect potential complications early, and provide personalized guidance for better disease management.

Here's why regular health screenings and check-ups are crucial for individuals with diabetes:

Early Detection of Complications:
  - Regular screenings help identify diabetes-related complications such as retinopathy, nephropathy, neuropathy, and cardiovascular diseases in their early stages.
  - Early detection allows for timely intervention and treatment, reducing the risk of complications progressing to more severe stages.

Blood Sugar Monitoring and Medication Adjustment:

- During check-ups, healthcare providers assess your blood sugar control through Hemoglobin A1c (HbA1c) tests and adjust medication regimens, if necessary, to optimize blood sugar levels.

- Monitoring blood sugar trends over time helps identify patterns and make appropriate changes to your diabetes management plan.

Blood Pressure and Cholesterol Management:

- Regular check-ups include monitoring blood pressure and cholesterol levels, important factors in reducing the risk of cardiovascular complications associated with diabetes.

- Healthcare providers can recommend lifestyle changes and medications to manage blood pressure and cholesterol effectively.

Kidney Function Tests:

- Routine kidney function tests, such as serum creatinine and urine albumin tests, assess kidney health and help detect early signs of diabetic nephropathy.

- Timely intervention can slow the progression of kidney disease and preserve kidney function.

Eye Examinations:

- Regular eye exams by an ophthalmologist or optometrist can identify diabetic retinopathy and other eye conditions related to diabetes.

- Early treatment can prevent vision loss and maintain eye health.

Foot Exams:

- Foot exams help detect potential foot complications, such as neuropathy and foot ulcers, which can arise due to reduced sensation and circulation associated with diabetes.

- Timely interventions and foot care guidance can prevent serious foot problems and lower the risk of amputation.

Individualized Diabetes Management Plan:

- Regular check-ups provide opportunities for open communication with healthcare providers about your diabetes management challenges and goals.

- Healthcare professionals can tailor your diabetes management plan based on your health status, lifestyle, and preferences.

Emotional and Psychological Support:

- Regular health check-ups offer opportunities to discuss the emotional and psychological aspects of living with diabetes.

- Healthcare providers can provide support, address emotional challenges, and refer individuals to counseling or support groups if needed.

Remember that regular health screenings and check-ups are not only about monitoring diabetes but also about comprehensive health assessments to identify potential issues early and ensure timely management. By maintaining regular appointments with your healthcare team, you can take proactive steps toward effective diabetes management, reduce the risk of complications, and improve your overall health and well-being.

CHAPTER 8: SUPPORT SYSTEMS AND RESOURCES

Living with diabetes can be made easier with the support of others and access to helpful resources. In this chapter, we explore the importance of finding diabetes support groups and communities, utilizing online resources and apps for diabetes management, and how family and friends can be a valuable source of support.

Finding Diabetes Support Groups and Communities

Diabetes support groups and communities play a crucial role in providing emotional support, camaraderie, and valuable insights for individuals living with diabetes. Connecting with others who understand the challenges of managing the condition can be empowering and uplifting. Here are some tips for finding diabetes support groups and communities:

Healthcare Provider Recommendations:

- Start by asking your healthcare provider, such as your primary care physician or endocrinologist, if they know of any local diabetes support groups. They may have information about community-based groups that meet regularly.

Diabetes Education Programs:

- Attend diabetes education programs or workshops organized by hospitals, clinics, or community centers. These programs often provide opportunities to connect with others who share similar experiences.

Online Resources and Social Media:

- Utilize online resources and social media platforms to find diabetes support groups and communities. Websites, forums, and social media groups dedicated to diabetes provide spaces for individuals to share their experiences, ask questions, and offer support to others.

National and International Diabetes Organizations:

- Check the websites of reputable diabetes organizations, such as the American Diabetes Association (ADA), Diabetes UK, or the International Diabetes Federation (IDF). These organizations often have information about local support groups or online communities.

Local Community Centers:

- Contact local community centers, libraries, or health organizations to inquire about any diabetes support groups they may host or know about in the area.

Ask Your Diabetes Educator:

- If you have a certified diabetes educator (CDE), ask them for recommendations on local support groups. They may be aware of community-based resources that can provide additional support and guidance.

Reach Out to Local Hospitals:

- Hospitals often offer support groups and workshops for individuals with diabetes. Contact the hospital's diabetes department or inquire at the patient resource center.

Meetup Groups:

- Explore meetup.com or other similar platforms to find diabetes-related meetups or support groups in your local area.

When joining a diabetes support group or community, consider the following:

- Check the group's focus and mission: Ensure that the group aligns with your needs and interests.

- Online vs. In-Person: Decide whether you prefer to join an online group or meet in-person for support meetings.
- Confidentiality: Ensure that the group respects members' privacy and maintains confidentiality regarding personal information shared.

Participating in diabetes support groups and communities can be a valuable addition to your diabetes management journey. Engaging with others who share similar experiences can provide emotional support, motivation, and practical insights for effectively managing diabetes and living a fulfilling life with the condition.

Utilizing Online Resources and Apps for Diabetes Management

With the advancement of technology, individuals with diabetes have access to a wide range of online resources and mobile apps that can significantly aid in diabetes management. These tools offer valuable support, tracking capabilities, and educational materials to help individuals effectively manage their condition. Here are some ways to utilize online resources and apps for diabetes management:

Diabetes Management Apps:

- Blood Sugar Tracking: Use mobile apps to log and track blood sugar levels regularly. These apps may provide visual trends and graphs to help identify patterns and make informed decisions about diabetes management.

- Medication Reminders: Set up medication reminders to ensure timely adherence to insulin injections, oral medications, or other diabetes-related medications.

- Food and Carb Tracking: Some apps have food databases that can help individuals track their carbohydrate intake and plan balanced meals.

- Physical Activity Monitoring: Use apps to record physical activity levels, track steps, and monitor exercise routines to promote an active lifestyle.

Nutrition and Recipe Apps:

- Utilize nutrition apps to access databases of food nutritional values, making it easier to plan diabetes-friendly meals and make informed food choices.

- Explore recipe apps that provide diabetes-friendly meal ideas, helping individuals maintain a healthy and varied diet.

Educational Websites:

- Visit reputable websites dedicated to diabetes education and management. These websites offer comprehensive information on topics such as meal planning, blood sugar management, and tips for living well with diabetes.

- Explore blogs and articles written by diabetes experts and individuals sharing their personal experiences and insights.

Continuous Glucose Monitoring (CGM) Apps:

- For individuals using CGM devices, apps are available that allow real-time tracking of blood sugar levels on smartphones, making it convenient to monitor glucose levels throughout the day.

Blood Pressure and Weight Tracking Apps:

- Some apps enable individuals to monitor and track blood pressure readings and weight, which are essential for overall health management, especially for those with diabetes.

Telemedicine and Virtual Visits:

- Utilize telemedicine platforms or virtual visits with healthcare providers for remote diabetes consultations, medication adjustments, and routine check-ins.

Online Diabetes Support Groups and Communities:

- Join online forums and social media groups dedicated to diabetes. Engaging with others who have diabetes can provide valuable support, motivation, and the exchange of practical tips for managing the condition.

When using online resources and apps for diabetes management, consider the following:

- Check for User Reviews: Read reviews and ratings before using an app or joining an online community to ensure it meets your needs and is reputable.
- Data Privacy and Security: Ensure that the app or online platform you use respects your data privacy and takes appropriate security measures to protect your information.

Remember that while online resources and apps can be valuable tools, they are meant to complement, not replace, professional medical advice. Always consult with your healthcare provider before making any significant changes to your diabetes management plan. By leveraging these digital tools effectively, individuals can gain better insights into their diabetes management, track progress, and receive support and educational resources that enhance their overall diabetes care.

Family and Friends as a Source of Support for Diabetes Management

The support of family and friends can play a crucial role in helping individuals with diabetes effectively manage their condition and cope with the challenges it presents. Their understanding, encouragement, and involvement can significantly improve the overall well-being of someone living with diabetes. Here are some ways in which family and friends can be a valuable source of support:

Emotional Support:

- Understanding and Empathy: Family and friends who are empathetic and understanding can provide a safe space for individuals with diabetes to express their feelings and concerns.

- Encouragement: Words of encouragement and positive reinforcement can boost confidence and motivation, especially during challenging times.

Practical Assistance:

- Meal Preparation: Loved ones can assist in preparing diabetes-friendly meals, making it easier for individuals to follow their meal plans and maintain a balanced diet.

- Exercise Buddy: Exercising together can be enjoyable and help ensure that individuals stay motivated to engage in regular physical activity.

- Medication Reminders: Family and friends can help with medication reminders, ensuring that individuals take their prescribed medications as directed.

Educating Themselves:

- Family and friends can educate themselves about diabetes to better understand the condition and how to provide appropriate support.

- Learning about diabetes management, dietary needs, and potential complications can help them actively participate in diabetes care.

Accompanying Medical Visits:

- Attending medical appointments with the individual can provide moral support and an extra set of ears during discussions with healthcare providers.

- Loved ones can also help ask questions and remember important instructions given by healthcare professionals.

Social Activities:

- Including individuals with diabetes in social activities and gatherings can help them feel included and supported in various settings.

- Friends and family can plan activities that align with the individual's dietary needs and encourage a healthy lifestyle.

Celebrating Achievements:

- Celebrating milestones and achievements in diabetes management, such as reaching blood sugar targets or maintaining a healthy weight, can reinforce positive behaviors and efforts.

Emergency Preparedness:

- Loved ones can be informed about what to do in case of a diabetes-related emergency, such as severe hypoglycemia (low blood sugar) or hyperglycemia (high blood sugar).

Open communication is key to building a strong support system. Individuals with diabetes should feel comfortable sharing their needs, preferences, and concerns with their family and friends. By openly discussing diabetes management and involving loved ones in the process, individuals can create a supportive environment that fosters their well-being and enhances their ability to manage diabetes effectively.

Additionally, it's essential for individuals with diabetes to recognize that support from family and friends is valuable, but they may also benefit from additional support networks, such as diabetes support groups or healthcare professionals specialized in diabetes care. By combining the support of loved ones with other resources, individuals can create a comprehensive and empowering approach to diabetes management.

CHAPTER 9: THRIVING WITH DIABETES: SUCCESS STORIES

In this chapter, we showcase inspiring success stories of individuals who have mastered diabetes, overcome challenges, and achieved personal goals while effectively managing their condition. These real-life accounts offer valuable lessons and insights into successful diabetes management, serving as a source of inspiration and encouragement for others facing similar challenges.

Inspirational Stories of People Who Have Mastered Diabetes

These inspirational stories highlight individuals who have successfully mastered diabetes and lead fulfilling lives while effectively managing their condition. Through determination, resilience, and a positive mindset, they have overcome challenges, achieved personal goals, and become shining examples of what it means to thrive with diabetes.

Lisa's Journey to Better Health:

- Lisa was diagnosed with type 2 diabetes and initially found it challenging to manage her blood sugar levels.

- She took charge of her health by making gradual lifestyle changes, including adopting a balanced diet and engaging in regular exercise.

- With the support of her family and healthcare team, Lisa lost weight, improved her blood sugar control, and experienced increased energy and overall well-being.

John's Marathon Triumph:

- John, a young man with type 1 diabetes, had a dream of running a marathon.

- He worked closely with his diabetes educator and endocrinologist to fine-tune his insulin regimen and manage blood sugar levels during training.

- Despite facing obstacles along the way, John completed his first marathon, proving that diabetes should not limit one's aspirations.

Maria's Advocacy for Diabetes Awareness:

- Maria was diagnosed with gestational diabetes during her pregnancy and later developed type 2 diabetes.

- She became an advocate for diabetes awareness, sharing her story to educate others about the importance of early detection and lifestyle modifications.

- Through her efforts, Maria has empowered many individuals to take control of their health and seek support for diabetes management.

David's Transformation with Technology:

- David, a tech-savvy individual with type 1 diabetes, embraced continuous glucose monitoring (CGM) technology.
- The data provided by the CGM enabled David to identify patterns in his blood sugar levels and fine-tune his insulin dosing effectively.
- With the help of the CGM and his healthcare team, David has achieved excellent blood sugar control and gained newfound confidence in managing his diabetes.

Sarah's Journey to Motherhood:

- Sarah had type 1 diabetes and desired to start a family.
- She worked closely with her healthcare providers to achieve optimal blood sugar control before conceiving.
- With meticulous planning and support, Sarah safely navigated her pregnancy, delivering a healthy baby, and became an inspiration to others with diabetes who dream of starting a family.

Mike's Positive Mindset and Personal Growth:

- Diagnosed with type 2 diabetes, Mike decided to view diabetes as an opportunity for personal growth.

- He embraced a healthy lifestyle, including regular exercise and mindful eating, and found joy in cooking diabetes-friendly meals.

- Through his positive attitude, Mike has not only improved his health but also enriched his life with new hobbies and passions.

These inspirational stories showcase the potential for individuals with diabetes to lead remarkable lives despite the challenges the condition presents. They remind us that diabetes management is not merely about adhering to treatment plans, but also about finding strength within, seeking support from loved ones and healthcare professionals, and maintaining a positive outlook. Each of these individuals has embraced their diabetes journey, transforming it from a perceived obstacle to a pathway for personal growth and empowerment. Their stories serve as beacons of hope and encouragement for others living with diabetes, inspiring them to believe in their own ability to thrive and achieve their goals.

Overcoming Challenges and Achieving Personal Goals

Living with diabetes presents unique challenges that require resilience, determination, and adaptability. Despite the obstacles, individuals with diabetes have shown incredible strength in overcoming these challenges and achieving personal goals.

Here are some inspiring examples of how people have triumphed over difficulties to accomplish their aspirations:

Blood Sugar Management for Athletic Pursuits:

- For individuals with type 1 diabetes who have a passion for sports or athletic pursuits, maintaining stable blood sugar levels during physical activities can be challenging.

- Through careful planning, frequent blood sugar monitoring, and close communication with healthcare providers, some athletes have successfully participated in marathons, triathlons, and other endurance events, proving that diabetes should not limit their athletic ambitions.

Pursuing Higher Education and Career Success:

- Diabetes management can be demanding, especially when juggling academic or professional responsibilities.

- Many individuals have persevered through their studies and careers, with proper time management, support from their academic institutions or employers, and a commitment to self-care.

Healthy Pregnancy and Parenthood:
 - For women with diabetes, planning and managing a healthy pregnancy require extra care and coordination with healthcare providers.
 - With diligent blood sugar control, nutritional guidance, and regular prenatal check-ups, many women with diabetes have successfully navigated pregnancy, giving birth to healthy babies.

Traveling and Adventure with Diabetes:
 - Individuals with diabetes have embarked on inspiring journeys around the world, managing their diabetes while exploring new cultures and environments.
 - Proper preparation, including packing essential supplies, adjusting insulin regimens for different time zones, and staying connected with healthcare providers, have empowered them to embark on adventures of a lifetime.

Advocacy and Diabetes Awareness:

- Some individuals have turned their diabetes journey into a platform for advocacy and raising awareness.

- By sharing their experiences and insights through public speaking, writing, or social media, they have inspired others, increased diabetes awareness, and promoted early detection and proper diabetes management.

Mental Health and Well-Being:

- Managing diabetes can have emotional and psychological impacts, requiring attention to mental health and well-being.

- Some individuals have embraced mindfulness practices, meditation, or counseling to cope with diabetes-related stress and maintain a positive mindset.

Achieving Weight Loss Goals:

- Weight management is a crucial aspect of diabetes management, especially for individuals with type 2 diabetes.

- Through commitment to healthier eating habits, regular exercise, and support from dietitians or weight management programs, many individuals have achieved significant weight loss, improving their diabetes control and overall health.

These stories of triumph highlight the power of determination, support systems, and a positive mindset in overcoming challenges and achieving personal goals. They demonstrate that diabetes management does not have to be a barrier to living life to the fullest and pursuing dreams. By taking control of their diabetes, seeking support, and embracing a proactive approach to self-care, individuals have proven that they can thrive and accomplish extraordinary feats. Their journeys serve as a beacon of hope and inspiration to others facing similar challenges, encouraging them to set ambitious goals, overcome obstacles, and lead fulfilling lives with diabetes.

Lessons and Insights from Successful Diabetes Management

Successful diabetes management involves a combination of knowledge, dedication, and the ability to adapt to changing circumstances. Individuals who have effectively managed their diabetes offer valuable lessons and insights that can benefit others on their diabetes journey. Here are some key lessons and insights from those who have achieved success in diabetes management:

Knowledge is Empowerment:

- Understanding diabetes and its management is crucial for effective control. Learn about the role of diet, exercise, medication, and blood sugar monitoring in diabetes care.

- Stay informed about new advancements in diabetes technology, treatment options, and lifestyle strategies to make informed decisions about your health.

Consistency in Blood Sugar Monitoring:

- Regularly monitoring blood sugar levels provides vital information about how various factors, such as food, exercise, stress, and medication, affect blood sugar.

- Consistent blood sugar monitoring empowers individuals to make timely adjustments to their diabetes management plan and maintain better control.

Individualized Approach:

- Diabetes management is not a one-size-fits-all approach. Customize your diabetes care plan based on your lifestyle, preferences, and unique needs.

- Work closely with your healthcare team to develop a personalized plan that aligns with your health goals and priorities.

Nutrition is Key:

- A balanced diet plays a crucial role in diabetes management. Focus on nutrient-rich foods, portion control, and mindful eating to manage blood sugar levels effectively.

- Choose a diet that is sustainable, enjoyable, and helps you maintain a healthy weight.

Regular Physical Activity:

- Incorporate regular exercise into your daily routine to improve insulin sensitivity, control blood sugar, and support overall health.

- Find physical activities that you enjoy to make exercise a positive and consistent part of your lifestyle.

Support System:

- Building a strong support system that includes family, friends, healthcare professionals, and diabetes support groups can make a significant difference in diabetes management.

- Seek encouragement, understanding, and practical assistance from your support network when needed.

Resilience and Adaptability:

- Diabetes management can be challenging and may involve setbacks. Embrace a resilient attitude and be open to adapting your approach as needed.

- Learn from challenges and use them as opportunities for growth and improvement in your diabetes management.

Mental Health Matters:

- Pay attention to your mental and emotional well-being. Diabetes can have an impact on mental health, so prioritize self-care and seek support if needed.

- Practice stress-reduction techniques, mindfulness, and seek professional help if you experience diabetes-related distress.

Advocacy and Empowerment:

- Become an advocate for yourself and others with diabetes. Empower yourself with knowledge and actively participate in your diabetes care decisions.

- Share your experiences to raise awareness, combat stigma, and inspire others in their diabetes journey.

Celebrate Progress:

- Celebrate your successes, no matter how small. Recognize the efforts you put into managing diabetes and celebrate the milestones you achieve.

- Positive reinforcement can strengthen your motivation and commitment to maintaining good diabetes control.

Remember that successful diabetes management is an ongoing journey that requires dedication and patience. By learning from those who have successfully managed their diabetes, individuals can gain valuable insights to help them lead healthier, happier lives while effectively managing their condition.

CHAPTER 10: EMBRACING A POSITIVE MINDSET

Maintaining a positive mindset is a powerful tool in diabetes management. In this chapter, we explore the impact of a positive attitude, setting realistic goals, and building resilience to navigate diabetes-related setbacks.

The Power of a Positive Attitude in Diabetes Management

A positive attitude can have a profound impact on diabetes management, shaping the way individuals approach their condition and the decisions they make in their daily lives. By embracing positivity, individuals can experience significant improvements in both their physical and emotional well-being. Here are some ways in which a positive attitude can empower individuals in diabetes management:

Enhanced Self-Efficacy: A positive attitude fosters a belief in one's ability to effectively manage diabetes. This sense of self-efficacy encourages individuals to take ownership of their health, adhere to their diabetes care plan, and face challenges with confidence.

Motivation and Adherence: A positive mindset motivates individuals to stay committed to their diabetes management routine. They are more likely to adhere to healthy habits, such as monitoring blood sugar levels, taking medications as prescribed, and maintaining a balanced diet.

Stress Reduction: A positive attitude can help reduce stress and anxiety associated with diabetes management. Managing stress is crucial, as it can impact blood sugar levels and overall well-being.

Resilience: A positive mindset equips individuals with the resilience to bounce back from setbacks and cope with diabetes-related challenges. Rather than being discouraged by obstacles, they see them as opportunities for growth and learning.

Improved Blood Sugar Control: Studies suggest that individuals with a positive outlook on diabetes management often experience improved blood sugar control compared to those with negative attitudes.

Better Communication with Healthcare Providers: A positive attitude can improve communication with healthcare providers, leading to more open and effective discussions about diabetes care, treatment options, and lifestyle adjustments.

Embracing Healthy Lifestyle Choices: A positive mindset encourages individuals to embrace healthy lifestyle choices willingly. They view these choices as acts of self-care and understand that they contribute to overall well-being.

Increased Social Support: Positivity attracts support from family, friends, and the diabetes community. A positive attitude can foster a strong support system that encourages and motivates individuals in their diabetes journey.

Reduced Diabetes-Related Distress: A positive attitude can reduce diabetes-related distress, which is essential for mental and emotional well-being. It helps individuals navigate the emotional challenges associated with diabetes effectively.

Mindfulness and Present-Moment Awareness: A positive attitude often goes hand in hand with mindfulness, promoting present-moment awareness and a non-judgmental approach to diabetes management.

It is essential to acknowledge that maintaining a positive attitude does not mean ignoring the challenges of living with diabetes. Rather, it is about approaching those challenges with optimism, seeking solutions, and focusing on progress rather than perfection. Embracing a positive mindset empowers individuals to take charge of their diabetes management and cultivate a sense of hope and possibility.

Practicing gratitude, setting realistic goals, and seeking support from loved ones and healthcare providers can further enhance the power of a positive attitude in diabetes management. By embracing positivity, individuals can transform their perspective on living with diabetes and create a foundation for a healthier and more fulfilling life with the condition.

Setting Realistic Goals and Celebrating Achievements in Diabetes Management

Setting realistic goals and celebrating achievements are essential components of effective diabetes management. By establishing achievable objectives and acknowledging progress, individuals can stay motivated, maintain a positive outlook, and experience greater success in their diabetes care journey. Here's how setting realistic goals and celebrating achievements contribute to diabetes management:

Focus on Incremental Progress: Setting realistic, achievable goals allows individuals to focus on incremental progress rather than overwhelming changes. Breaking down larger goals into smaller, manageable steps makes it easier to stay on track and maintain motivation.

Define Measurable Objectives: Clearly define goals that are measurable and specific. For example, aiming to reduce HbA1c levels by a certain percentage or tracking daily physical activity minutes are tangible and measurable objectives.

Empowerment and Ownership: Setting personal goals empowers individuals to take ownership of their diabetes management. It instills a sense of control and responsibility, fostering a proactive approach to care.

Celebrate Small Victories: Celebrating even minor achievements along the diabetes management journey is vital. Recognizing small victories, such as consistent blood sugar readings or achieving daily exercise goals, boosts self-esteem and reinforces positive behaviors.

Reinforce Positive Behaviors: Celebrating achievements reinforces positive behaviors and encourages individuals to continue making healthy choices. Positive reinforcement increases the likelihood of maintaining beneficial habits.

Boost Motivation: Acknowledging progress and celebrating achievements can be motivating. It encourages individuals to continue working towards their goals and overcome any obstacles they may encounter.

Build Resilience: Celebrating achievements builds resilience, as it emphasizes progress rather than perfection. It fosters a growth mindset and helps individuals bounce back from setbacks with determination.

Share Successes with Support Network: Celebrating achievements with family, friends, or a diabetes support group strengthens the support network and creates a positive, encouraging environment.

Evaluate and Adjust: Celebrating achievements provides an opportunity to evaluate the effectiveness of the current diabetes management plan. If goals are consistently met, individuals can discuss with their healthcare provider the possibility of adjusting treatment plans to maintain progress.

Set New Challenges: Celebrating achievements paves the way for setting new, challenging goals. As individuals accomplish their objectives, they can aim for higher targets to continue improving their diabetes management.

It's essential to remember that diabetes management is a continuous journey. Setting realistic goals and celebrating achievements along the way is an ongoing process that promotes consistent progress and positive change. Celebrating both small and significant accomplishments contributes to an optimistic mindset, making diabetes management feel less burdensome and more rewarding.

When celebrating achievements, individuals can engage in various activities, such as rewarding themselves with non-food-related treats, sharing successes with loved ones, journaling progress, or participating in diabetes-related events or communities. By celebrating the successes achieved through diligent diabetes management, individuals reinforce their commitment to self-care, boost confidence, and lay the foundation for a healthier and fulfilling life with diabetes.

Building Resilience in the Face of Diabetes-Related Setbacks

Living with diabetes involves managing various challenges, and setbacks are an inevitable part of the journey. Building resilience is crucial for effectively navigating these obstacles and maintaining a positive outlook on diabetes management. Resilience empowers individuals to bounce back from setbacks, adapt to changes, and continue their commitment to self-care. Here are some strategies for building resilience in the face of diabetes-related setbacks:

Embrace a Growth Mindset: Adopt a growth mindset that views setbacks as opportunities for learning and growth. Instead of viewing setbacks as failures, see them as stepping stones to better diabetes management.

Seek Support: Reach out to your support network, including family, friends, and healthcare providers, when facing setbacks. Sharing your challenges and feelings can provide emotional support and perspective.

Self-Compassion: Be kind to yourself and practice self-compassion. Acknowledge that setbacks are a natural part of life, and it's okay to experience frustration or disappointment. Treat yourself with the same kindness and understanding you would offer to a friend facing a similar situation.

Focus on What You Can Control: Recognize that not everything in diabetes management is within your control. Concentrate on the aspects of your care that you can influence, such as adhering to medication regimens, making healthy lifestyle choices, and monitoring blood sugar levels.

Learn from Setbacks: Use setbacks as opportunities for self-reflection and learning. Identify factors that contributed to the setback and consider adjustments to your diabetes management plan that could prevent similar situations in the future.

Set Realistic Expectations: Set achievable goals and expectations for yourself in diabetes management. Unrealistic expectations can lead to disappointment and feelings of inadequacy.

Mindfulness and Stress Reduction: Practice mindfulness techniques and stress reduction strategies to cope with feelings of overwhelm and anxiety caused by setbacks.

Mindfulness helps maintain focus on the present moment and reduces the impact of negative emotions.

Maintain a Positive Support System: Surround yourself with a positive support system that encourages and uplifts you. Engage in support groups or online communities of individuals with diabetes to share experiences and gain insight from others facing similar challenges.

Celebrate Resilience: Recognize and celebrate your resilience in overcoming setbacks. Acknowledge your strength and ability to persevere in diabetes management, even in the face of challenges.

Remember Past Achievements: Reflect on past successes and achievements in diabetes management. Remind yourself of the progress you have made, and draw strength from those accomplishments to face new setbacks.

Building resilience is a continuous process that strengthens over time with practice and perseverance. Developing coping skills and a positive mindset empowers individuals to navigate the ups and downs of diabetes management with confidence and determination. Resilience is not about avoiding challenges, but rather about developing the ability to adapt, learn, and grow in the face of adversity. By cultivating resilience, individuals can maintain a sense of empowerment, optimism, and overall well-being on their diabetes journey.

CHAPTER 11: LIVING YOUR BEST LIFE WITH DIABETES

Living a fulfilling life with diabetes involves striking a balance between effective diabetes management and pursuing personal interests and passions. In this chapter, we explore strategies for achieving this balance, embracing a sense of purpose, and empowering oneself to lead a vibrant life with diabetes.

Strategies for Balancing Diabetes Management and a Fulfilling Life

Achieving a balance between effective diabetes management and leading a fulfilling life is essential for overall well-being and happiness. Successfully integrating diabetes care into daily routines while pursuing personal interests and goals can contribute to a vibrant and satisfying life. Here are some strategies to help you strike a harmonious balance:

Develop a Flexible Diabetes Care Plan:

- Create a diabetes care plan that is adaptable to your lifestyle and individual needs. Consider factors like work schedule, social activities, and hobbies when planning your diabetes management routine.

Set Realistic Diabetes Goals:

- Establish achievable diabetes management goals that align with your overall life priorities. Avoid setting overly ambitious targets that may lead to frustration.

Prioritize Self-Care:

- Make self-care a priority by incorporating time for relaxation, exercise, and other activities that promote physical and emotional well-being.

- Recognize that taking care of yourself is crucial for effectively managing diabetes and enjoying life to the fullest.

Time Management:

- Practice effective time management to balance diabetes tasks, work, family, and leisure activities.

- Use calendars, reminders, and task lists to stay organized and ensure that diabetes care is integrated seamlessly into your daily schedule.

Embrace Mindfulness:

- Practice mindfulness to stay present in the moment and fully engage in daily activities without feeling overwhelmed by diabetes management.
- Mindfulness can reduce stress and enhance your overall well-being.

Involve Loved Ones:
- Involve your family and friends in your diabetes management journey. Communicate openly about your needs and seek their support and understanding.
- Share your achievements and challenges with loved ones to foster a sense of connection and encouragement.

Pursue Diabetes-Friendly Hobbies:
- Explore hobbies and interests that align with your diabetes management goals. Engaging in physical activities, arts, or other enjoyable pursuits can enhance your overall well-being.

Seek Professional Guidance:
- Work closely with your healthcare team to develop a diabetes care plan that fits your lifestyle and aspirations.
- Regularly consult with your healthcare provider to make adjustments to your diabetes management as needed.

Set Boundaries:

- Establish boundaries to prevent diabetes from dominating your life. Allocate time for self-care, relaxation, and activities unrelated to diabetes.

- Communicate your boundaries to others, advocating for your need to balance diabetes management with other aspects of life.

Celebrate Achievements:

- Celebrate your diabetes management milestones and accomplishments, no matter how small. Recognize and reward yourself for progress and achievements along the way.

Striking a balance between diabetes management and a fulfilling life requires ongoing effort and self-awareness. Remember that it's okay to seek support from loved ones, healthcare providers, or diabetes support groups when facing challenges. By adopting a proactive and positive approach to diabetes management, you can cultivate a fulfilling life that integrates diabetes care with your passions and goals. A balanced approach empowers you to embrace life's opportunities, find joy in your journey, and thrive with diabetes.

Pursuing Hobbies, Interests, and Passions with Diabetes

Having diabetes does not mean giving up on hobbies, interests, and passions. In fact, embracing and actively engaging in activities that bring joy and fulfillment can enhance overall well-being and complement diabetes management. With thoughtful planning and consideration, individuals with diabetes can continue to enjoy their favorite hobbies and explore new interests. Here are some strategies for pursuing hobbies, interests, and passions while effectively managing diabetes:

Consult with Healthcare Providers:

- Before starting or resuming a hobby or physical activity, consult with your healthcare provider. Discuss any potential risks, and ensure that your diabetes care plan is tailored to accommodate your chosen activity.

Choose Diabetes-Friendly Hobbies:

- Opt for hobbies and interests that align well with your diabetes management goals. Consider activities that promote physical fitness, such as walking, swimming, or gardening, which can positively impact blood sugar levels.

Be Prepared with Supplies:

- Carry essential diabetes supplies, such as glucose monitoring devices, insulin, snacks, and water, when participating in activities outside your home.

- Stay attentive to blood sugar levels during activities that may affect glucose levels.

Snack Smartly:

- If your hobby involves physical exertion, be prepared with diabetes-friendly snacks to prevent low blood sugar episodes.

- Keep a supply of quick-acting carbohydrates, like glucose tablets or juice, on hand to treat hypoglycemia promptly.

Stay Hydrated:

- Hydration is essential for overall health and diabetes management. Stay hydrated during physical activities and hobbies that may cause increased perspiration.

Listen to Your Body:

- Pay attention to how your body responds to different activities. Take breaks when needed, and be mindful of signs of fatigue or fluctuations in blood sugar levels.

Join Diabetes-Friendly Groups:

- Explore diabetes-friendly clubs or support groups related to your interests or hobbies. Connecting with others who share similar passions can offer camaraderie and encouragement.

Use Technology for Support:

- Utilize diabetes apps or wearable devices to track blood sugar levels, physical activity, and nutrition. These tools can provide valuable insights and help you manage diabetes while enjoying your hobbies.

Set Realistic Goals:

- Set achievable goals related to your hobbies and interests, taking your diabetes management into account.
- Remember that progress may be gradual, but each step forward is a testament to your commitment and determination.

Celebrate Successes:

- Celebrate your achievements and milestones in both diabetes management and your hobbies. Recognize and reward yourself for progress, whether in blood sugar control or mastering a new hobby skill.

Pursuing hobbies, interests, and passions is a vital aspect of maintaining a fulfilling life with diabetes. Engaging in enjoyable activities can reduce stress, increase happiness, and promote emotional well-being. Remember that diabetes management should not hold you back from living life to the fullest. By integrating your passions and diabetes care, you can create a balanced and enriching lifestyle that positively impacts both your physical and mental health.

Embracing a Sense of Purpose and Self-Empowerment with Diabetes

Embracing a sense of purpose and self-empowerment is essential for individuals living with diabetes. Developing a clear purpose and cultivating a positive mindset empowers individuals to take charge of their diabetes management, make informed decisions, and lead a fulfilling life. Here are ways to embrace a sense of purpose and self-empowerment with diabetes:

Define Your Purpose:

- Reflect on what matters most to you and what brings meaning to your life. Consider how diabetes management aligns with your personal values and life goals.

- Identifying your purpose in diabetes care can provide motivation and a sense of direction.

Take Ownership of Your Diabetes:

- Acknowledge that you are the primary advocate for your health. Take an active role in managing your diabetes and be proactive in your care decisions.
- Empower yourself with knowledge about diabetes, treatment options, and lifestyle strategies.

Set Personal Health Goals:

- Establish specific, achievable health goals related to your diabetes management. Breaking down larger goals into smaller steps makes progress more manageable.
- Monitor your progress and celebrate achievements along the way.

Practice Positive Self-Talk:

- Cultivate a positive inner dialogue and avoid self-criticism or negative thoughts related to diabetes management.
- Replace self-doubt with affirmations that reinforce your capabilities and resilience.

Learn from Setbacks:

- View setbacks as opportunities for growth and learning. Accept that challenges are a natural part of managing diabetes and that it's okay to encounter obstacles.

- Analyze setbacks objectively, identify potential solutions, and use them as valuable lessons for future decisions.

Seek Support:

- Surround yourself with a supportive network of family, friends, and healthcare providers who understand and encourage your efforts in diabetes management.

- Share your diabetes journey with others who have similar experiences through support groups or online communities.

Advocate for Yourself:

- Be your own advocate when it comes to your diabetes care. Communicate openly with healthcare providers about your preferences and concerns.

- Take an active role in treatment decisions and work collaboratively with your healthcare team.

Embrace Resilience:

- Embrace resilience as a key attribute in managing diabetes. Resilience helps you bounce back from setbacks, maintain a positive outlook, and persevere in your health journey.

Focus on Progress, Not Perfection:
  - Shift your mindset from striving for perfection to recognizing progress and efforts in diabetes management. Avoid self-criticism for not being "perfect" and celebrate each step forward.

Engage in Activities that Bring Joy:
  - Engage in activities that bring joy and fulfillment, whether related to diabetes management or unrelated hobbies and interests.
  - Find a sense of purpose beyond diabetes care by pursuing your passions and engaging in activities that enrich your life.

By embracing a sense of purpose and self-empowerment, individuals with diabetes can foster a positive mindset, make informed decisions, and maintain a strong commitment to their health. With determination and resilience, it is possible to lead a fulfilling life with diabetes, achieving physical and emotional well-being while pursuing meaningful goals and aspirations. Remember that every step taken towards self-empowerment contributes to a healthier and more purposeful life with diabetes.

CHAPTER 12: THE FUTURE OF DIABETES MANAGEMENT

In this chapter, we delve into the exciting developments and advancements in diabetes research, technology, and treatment options. By exploring the potential for groundbreaking innovations and the importance of staying informed, individuals can look forward to a brighter future in diabetes management.

Exploring Advancements in Diabetes Research and Technology

Advancements in diabetes research and technology have transformed diabetes management, providing individuals with innovative tools and solutions to better control their condition and improve their quality of life. In this chapter, we delve into the exciting developments that are shaping the future of diabetes care:

Continuous Glucose Monitoring (CGM):

- CGM technology enables real-time monitoring of glucose levels, providing valuable data to help individuals

121

make informed decisions about their insulin dosing, diet, and physical activity.

- CGM systems offer alerts for high and low blood sugar levels, allowing for prompt action to prevent extreme fluctuations.

Closed-Loop Systems (Artificial Pancreas):

- Closed-loop systems, also known as artificial pancreas systems, automate insulin delivery based on CGM readings.

- These systems reduce the burden of constant monitoring and provide a more seamless approach to insulin management, improving overall glycemic control.

Smart Insulin Pens and Patch Pumps:

- Smart insulin pens and patch pumps offer more convenient insulin delivery options, making it easier for individuals to manage their insulin dosing discreetly and efficiently.

- These devices often integrate with smartphone apps, allowing for data tracking and remote monitoring.

Advanced Insulin Analogues:

- Ongoing research has led to the development of faster-acting insulins and long-acting insulins with improved pharmacokinetics.

- Advanced insulin analogues offer better glycemic control and flexibility in managing mealtimes and insulin doses.

Personalized Medicine and Precision Therapy:

- The concept of personalized medicine tailors diabetes management to individual needs, genetics, and lifestyle factors.

- Precision therapy aims to identify specific molecular targets for treating diabetes more effectively and with fewer side effects.

Artificial Intelligence (AI) and Data Analytics:

- AI and data analytics play a crucial role in diabetes research and management, analyzing large datasets to identify patterns and trends in blood glucose fluctuations.

- AI-driven algorithms help optimize insulin dosing and predict potential hypoglycemic or hyperglycemic events.

Advanced Beta-Cell Replacement Therapies:

- Researchers are exploring innovative approaches to replace or regenerate beta cells in the pancreas, which produce insulin.

- Beta-cell replacement therapies hold the potential to restore insulin production in individuals with type 1 diabetes.

Stem Cell Research:

- Stem cell research explores the possibility of using stem cells to regenerate insulin-producing beta cells.

- This research has promising implications for both type 1 and type 2 diabetes treatment.

Gene Editing Technologies:

- Gene editing technologies, such as CRISPR-Cas9, offer possibilities for correcting genetic mutations that contribute to diabetes.

- These technologies have the potential to address the root causes of certain forms of diabetes.

Telemedicine and Remote Monitoring:

- Telemedicine and remote monitoring have become integral to diabetes care, allowing healthcare providers to monitor patients' glucose levels and offer support remotely.

- Virtual consultations and digital health platforms enhance accessibility and patient-provider communication.

Exploring advancements in diabetes research and technology provides hope for a future where diabetes management is more efficient, personalized, and effective. Staying informed about these developments empowers individuals to make well-informed decisions about their diabetes care and take advantage of the latest tools and treatments available. As technology continues to evolve, individuals with diabetes can look forward to a brighter future with enhanced support and improved overall well-being.

Promising Treatments and Potential Cures on the Horizon for Diabetes

In recent years, significant progress has been made in diabetes research, offering promising treatments and potential cures on the horizon. These developments provide hope for individuals living with diabetes and those at risk of developing the condition. While a complete cure for diabetes is yet to be achieved, ongoing research is opening new avenues for improved diabetes management and the possibility of long-term solutions. Here are some of the promising treatments and potential cures that hold great potential for the future:

Beta-Cell Replacement Therapies:

 - Beta-cell replacement therapies aim to restore insulin-producing beta cells in individuals with type 1 diabetes. These therapies include islet cell transplantation and stem cell-based approaches.

- Researchers are exploring ways to protect transplanted beta cells from immune attacks to achieve long-lasting insulin independence.

Stem Cell Therapy:

- Stem cell research shows promise in regenerating damaged beta cells or producing insulin-secreting cells, potentially benefiting individuals with both type 1 and type 2 diabetes.

- By harnessing the regenerative capabilities of stem cells, researchers hope to find ways to replace damaged or lost beta cells, leading to improved glycemic control.

Immunotherapies:

- Immunotherapies focus on modulating the immune system to prevent the destruction of insulin-producing beta cells in type 1 diabetes.

- Research in this area aims to halt or slow down the autoimmune process that leads to the development of type 1 diabetes.

Gene Editing Technologies:

- Gene editing technologies, such as CRISPR-Cas9, hold the potential to correct genetic mutations associated with certain forms of diabetes.

- By precisely targeting and editing genes, researchers aim to address the root causes of monogenic diabetes and other genetic forms of the condition.

Encapsulation Technology:

- Encapsulation technology involves creating protective barriers around transplanted beta cells to shield them from the immune system's attack.

- These encapsulation devices aim to provide long-term insulin independence while minimizing the need for immunosuppressive medications.

Glucose-Responsive Insulin:

- Glucose-responsive insulin seeks to develop insulin formulations that automatically adjust their activity in response to blood sugar levels.

- This technology aims to mimic the natural insulin release seen in people without diabetes, leading to improved glucose control and reduced risk of hypoglycemia.

Artificial Pancreas and Closed-Loop Systems:

- Artificial pancreas and closed-loop systems combine continuous glucose monitoring with automated insulin delivery.

- These advanced systems aim to optimize insulin dosing and provide a more seamless and automated approach to diabetes management.

Diabetes Vaccines:

- Diabetes vaccines are being explored as a potential preventive measure for type 1 diabetes, aimed at stopping the autoimmune process that destroys beta cells.

- These vaccines could be administered to individuals at high risk of developing type 1 diabetes to protect their remaining beta cells.

While these treatments and potential cures offer hope for the future of diabetes management, it's essential to recognize that research is still ongoing, and further clinical trials and validation are required to ensure their safety and effectiveness. Nonetheless, the progress made in these areas inspires optimism and fuels the dedication of researchers, healthcare professionals, and individuals affected by diabetes worldwide. As research continues to advance, the outlook for diabetes management and potential cures becomes increasingly promising, offering a brighter future for those living with diabetes.

The Importance of Staying Informed and Engaged in the Diabetes Community

Staying informed and engaged in the diabetes community is vital for individuals living with diabetes, their families, and caregivers. Diabetes is a complex and ever-evolving condition, and being proactive in staying informed offers numerous benefits for effectively managing the condition and improving overall well-being. Here are some key reasons why staying informed and engaged in the diabetes community is essential:

Access to the Latest Information:

- Diabetes research and treatment options are constantly evolving. Staying informed keeps individuals updated on the latest advancements in diabetes management, technology, and potential cures.

- Access to up-to-date information allows individuals to make well-informed decisions about their treatment plans and lifestyle choices.

Empowerment and Self-Advocacy:

- Knowledge is empowering. When individuals understand their condition, treatment options, and the latest research, they become active participants in their diabetes care.

- Staying informed enables individuals to advocate for themselves during healthcare appointments and make informed choices about their diabetes management.

Community Support and Connection:

- Engaging with the diabetes community offers a sense of belonging and support. Interacting with others who share similar experiences fosters understanding, empathy, and emotional support.

- The diabetes community provides a safe space to share challenges, triumphs, and practical tips for managing the condition.

Learning from Others' Experiences:

- Within the diabetes community, individuals can learn from the experiences of others who have faced similar challenges and triumphs in managing diabetes.

- Learning from others' journeys can offer valuable insights, coping strategies, and inspiration.

Access to Peer Support:

- Diabetes support groups and online forums provide opportunities to connect with peers who understand the day-to-day realities of living with diabetes.

- Peer support can alleviate feelings of isolation and provide encouragement during difficult times.

Improved Diabetes Management:

- Being informed about diabetes management strategies, dietary guidelines, and exercise recommendations enhances one's ability to control blood sugar levels effectively.

- Staying informed helps individuals identify potential barriers to good diabetes management and find solutions for overcoming them.

Advocacy and Awareness:

- Being engaged in the diabetes community allows individuals to participate in advocacy efforts, raise awareness about diabetes, and promote understanding of the condition.

- Advocacy helps drive policy changes, improve access to healthcare, and increase research funding for diabetes.

Emotional Well-Being:

- Understanding the complexities of diabetes and having a support network positively impact emotional well-being and mental health.

- Being informed and engaged can reduce stress and anxiety related to diabetes management.

Opportunities for Education:

- Participation in diabetes education programs and workshops provides valuable insights into self-care, nutrition, physical activity, and medication management.

- Education empowers individuals to take control of their diabetes and make lifestyle changes that improve their health.

Awareness of Clinical Trials and Research Studies:

- Staying informed about ongoing clinical trials and research studies allows individuals to explore potential participation in cutting-edge research for diabetes treatment and cures.

By staying informed and engaged in the diabetes community, individuals can actively participate in their diabetes management, access valuable resources, and foster a sense of support and connection. Empowered by knowledge and community support, individuals can navigate the challenges of diabetes with confidence and strive for a healthier and more fulfilling life.

CONCLUSION

As we reach the conclusion of "From Diagnosis to Control: Mastering Diabetes for a Better Life," we reflect on the journey of empowerment and resilience that individuals with diabetes and their loved ones have embarked upon. Throughout this book, we have explored the multifaceted aspects of diabetes, delving into understanding the condition, mastering diabetes management, and embracing a positive mindset for a fulfilling life.

Diabetes is a formidable challenge, but it is one that can be met with determination, knowledge, and support. From the moment of diagnosis, we have emphasized the importance of understanding the different types of diabetes, the causes and risk factors, and the role of insulin and blood sugar regulation. Armed with this knowledge, individuals can make informed decisions and actively participate in their diabetes care.

In subsequent chapters, we explored lifestyle changes, nutrition, physical activity, and blood sugar monitoring as essential pillars of diabetes management. Recognizing the significance of pursuing hobbies, interests, and passions while managing diabetes, we encouraged a balanced approach to life that integrates diabetes care seamlessly into daily routines.

The book also shed light on the emotional and psychological aspects of diabetes, addressing stress, burnout, and peer pressure. By fostering a positive mindset, setting realistic goals, and building resilience, individuals can overcome challenges and celebrate their achievements on the path to better diabetes control.

Throughout these pages, we explored advancements in diabetes research, technology, and potential cures on the horizon. While we are on the cusp of remarkable breakthroughs, we highlighted the importance of staying informed and engaged in the diabetes community to take advantage of new tools, treatments, and support systems.

As we conclude this journey, we recognize that diabetes is not just a medical condition; it is a way of life. Empowered by knowledge, connected through community, and embracing a sense of purpose, individuals can master diabetes for a better life. This book serves as a guiding light, empowering readers to take charge of their diabetes care, advocate for themselves, and find strength and support in the diabetes community.

Remember, you are not alone on this journey. Together, we will navigate the complexities of diabetes, celebrate triumphs, and find hope in the advancements of science. By embracing a positive mindset, nurturing resilience, and staying informed, individuals can thrive with diabetes and lead a fulfilling life.

As the author, I hope that "From Diagnosis to Control: Mastering Diabetes for a Better Life" becomes a companion, offering guidance, knowledge, and inspiration in your diabetes journey. May this book empower you to embrace your potential, embrace a life of wellness and purpose, and embrace the possibilities that lie ahead. Remember, diabetes may be a part of your life, but it does not define you. With knowledge, perseverance, and the support of the diabetes community, you can master diabetes for a better life. Wishing you health, happiness, and success on this transformative path ahead.